Embracing Balance:

Living with Borderline Personality Disorder

Mark Winters

Embracing Balance: Living with Borderline Personality
Disorder

Author Mark Winters

Published By Neil McKenzie

ISBN 9781445274010
Imprint: Lulu.com

Chapter 1.

Understanding Borderline Personality Disorder

- Symptoms, causes, and common misconceptions.

Chapter 2.

Diagnosis and Acceptance

- Coping with the initial diagnosis and coming to terms with living with BPD.

Chapter 3.

Building a Support System

- The importance of supportive relationships and finding understanding.

Chapter 4.

Cognitive Behavioural Strategies

  - Practical techniques for managing intense emotions and impulsivity.

Chapter 5.

Dialectical Behaviour Therapy

  - Explanation of DBT principles and how they can be applied in daily life.

Chapter 6.

Mindfulness and Grounding Techniques

  - Exercises to stay present and manage dissociation.

Chapter 7.

Navigating Relationships

- How BPD affects relationships and strategies for healthier interactions.

Chapter 8.

Self-Care and Well-being

- Importance of self-care practices and developing a routine that supports mental health.

Chapter 9.

Setting Boundaries

- Learning to set and maintain boundaries to protect emotional well-being.

Chapter 10.

Personal Growth and Recovery

- Stories of hope, resilience, and personal growth from individuals with BPD.

Finding Light at the End of the Tunnel: Hope and Help for Those with BPD

Chapter 1.

Understanding Borderline Personality Disorder

- Symptoms, causes, and common misconceptions.

Understanding Borderline Personality Disorder

Borderline Personality Disorder (BPD) is a multifaceted mental health condition that affects how a person thinks, feels, and interacts with others. Often characterised by intense emotional experiences, impulsivity, and unstable relationships, BPD can profoundly influence every aspect of a person's life.

The Emotional Rollercoaster

Imagine feeling like you're constantly on an emotional rollercoaster, where every peak and valley is amplified beyond measure. For individuals with BPD, emotions can be overwhelmingly intense and change rapidly. What may seem like a minor setback to others can trigger a tidal wave of despair or rage. This emotional volatility can lead to impulsive behaviours such as reckless spending, substance abuse, or self-harm—desperate attempts to cope with inner turmoil.

Fear of Abandonment

At the core of BPD often lies a deep-seated fear of abandonment. This fear can manifest in frantic efforts to avoid real or imagined abandonment, even in the face of stable relationships. Individuals with BPD may go to great lengths to maintain connections, yet perceive rejection where none exists. This fear can strain relationships and reinforce a cycle of emotional instability.

Identity Disturbance

Another hallmark of BPD is a profound disturbance in self-image and identity. Individuals may struggle with an unstable sense of self, uncertain of their values, goals, or even their own personality. This instability can lead to feelings of emptiness and a chronic sense of dissatisfaction or boredom with life.

Challenges in Relationships

Navigating relationships can be particularly challenging for those with BPD. Interpersonal relationships are often marked by extremes—idealisation and intense attachment one moment, followed by devaluation and conflict the next. This pattern, known as "splitting," can strain relationships and contribute to a cycle of tumultuous interactions.

The Role of Trauma

While the exact causes of BPD are not fully understood, research suggests that a combination of genetic predisposition, neurobiological factors, and early life experiences—such as trauma or invalidating environments—may contribute to its development. These factors can shape emotional regulation skills and coping mechanisms, influencing how individuals with BPD respond to stressors.

Treatment and Hope

Despite its challenges, BPD is treatable. Dialectical Behaviour Therapy (DBT) has emerged as one of the most effective therapeutic approaches, emphasising mindfulness, emotion regulation, interpersonal effectiveness, and distress tolerance skills. Therapy can provide individuals with BPD the tools to manage intense emotions, improve relationships, and cultivate a stronger sense of self.

Breaking the Stigma

Understanding BPD is essential in breaking down stigma and promoting compassion and support for those affected. It's important to recognise that BPD does not define a person; rather, it is one aspect of their complex and unique identity. With understanding, empathy, and effective treatment, individuals with BPD can lead fulfilling lives and build meaningful connections.

Borderline personality disorder is a complex mental health condition that deserves nuanced understanding and compassionate support. By raising awareness and providing effective treatment options, we can create a more inclusive and supportive environment for individuals living with BPD.

Symptoms, causes, and common misconceptions

Borderline Personality Disorder (BPD) is a deeply misunderstood mental health condition characterised by pervasive patterns of instability in mood, interpersonal relationships, self-image, and behaviour. Despite its prevalence and impact, BPD often remains shrouded in misconceptions and stigma. Let's delve into the symptoms, causes, and common misconceptions surrounding BPD to foster a clearer understanding.

Symptoms of Borderline Personality Disorder

1. Emotional Instability:

   - Individuals with BPD often experience intense, unstable emotions that can fluctuate rapidly. They may feel intense happiness, sadness, or anger within short periods, sometimes triggered by seemingly minor events.

2. Fear of Abandonment:

- There is a persistent fear of abandonment and a frantic effort to avoid real or imagined separation from loved ones. This fear can lead to clinginess, drastic measures to avoid being alone, or dramatic responses to perceived rejection.

3. Unstable Relationships:

- Relationships are characterised by extremes of idealisation and devaluation, known as "splitting." People with BPD may idolise someone one moment and demonise them the next, causing turmoil and instability in their interpersonal connections.

4. Distorted Self-Image:

- Individuals with BPD often struggle with a distorted sense of self and identity. They may experience uncertainty about their values, goals, career choices, or even their sexual orientation.

5. Impulsive Behaviours:

   - Impulsivity is common in BPD, manifesting in reckless behaviours such as substance abuse, binge eating, reckless driving, or risky sexual encounters. These behaviours are often attempts to alleviate emotional pain or seek validation.

6. Self-Harm or Suicidal Behaviour:

   - People with BPD may engage in self-harming behaviours such as cutting or burning themselves as a way to cope with overwhelming emotions. Suicidal thoughts, threats, or attempts are also prevalent, particularly during times of extreme distress.

7. Chronic Feelings of Emptiness:

   - Many individuals with BPD report feeling empty, bored, or devoid of emotions. This persistent feeling of emptiness can drive them to seek stimulation or engage in impulsive behaviours to fill the void.

8. Intense Anger:

 - Frequent displays of intense anger or difficulty
controlling anger are common in BPD. These outbursts
may be triggered by perceived criticism or rejection,
contributing to interpersonal conflicts.

Causes of Borderline Personality Disorder

1. Biological Factors:

 - Research suggests that genetics and family history
may play a role in predisposing individuals to BPD.
Differences in brain structure and function, particularly
in areas that regulate emotions and impulse control, have
also been observed.

2. Environmental Factors:

 - Early life experiences such as trauma, neglect, or
unstable relationships during childhood can significantly
increase the risk of developing BPD. These experiences

may disrupt the development of healthy coping mechanisms and emotional regulation skills.

3. Neurobiological Factors:

 - Dysregulation in neurotransmitters, particularly serotonin and dopamine, has been implicated in the emotional dysregulation and impulsivity seen in BPD. Imbalances in these neurotransmitters may contribute to the intense mood swings and impulsive behaviours characteristic of the disorder.

Common Misconceptions about Borderline Personality Disorder

1. BPD is Attention-Seeking Behaviour:

 - Contrary to popular belief, behaviours associated with BPD, such as self-harm or suicidal gestures, are often desperate attempts to cope with overwhelming emotional pain rather than mere attention-seeking.

2. People with BPD Cannot Maintain Stable Relationships:

- While relationships may be tumultuous due to the instability associated with BPD, individuals with the disorder can form and maintain meaningful relationships with appropriate support and therapy.

3. BPD is Rare:

- BPD is more common than often perceived, with prevalence estimates ranging from 1.6% to 5.9% in the general population. It affects men and women equally and can occur across all ethnic and socioeconomic backgrounds.

4. BPD is Untreatable:

- With appropriate treatment and support, individuals with BPD can experience significant improvement in symptoms and lead fulfilling lives. Dialectical Behaviour Therapy (DBT), Cognitive Behavioural Therapy (CBT), and medications can be effective in managing symptoms.

5. BPD is the Same as Bipolar Disorder:

- While both disorders involve mood instability, BPD and Bipolar Disorder are distinct conditions with different diagnostic criteria, causes, and treatment approaches.

Borderline Personality Disorder is a complex and challenging mental health condition that requires compassionate understanding, accurate information, and effective treatment approaches. By dispelling misconceptions and promoting awareness, we can create a more supportive environment for individuals living with BPD, fostering hope and recovery.

Chapter 2.

Diagnosis and Acceptance

- Coping with the initial diagnosis and coming to terms with living with BPD.

Diagnosis and Acceptance

Receiving a diagnosis of borderline personality disorder (BPD) can be a pivotal moment in one's life—a moment filled with confusion, relief, and often, a profound sense of validation. Understanding the journey of diagnosis and acceptance is crucial in navigating the complexities of BPD and embarking on a path toward healing and self-understanding.

The Road to Diagnosis

1. Recognition of Symptoms:

- For many individuals, the journey begins with the recognition of persistent patterns of emotional instability, turbulent relationships, and difficulties in self-image and identity. Symptoms such as intense mood swings, fear of abandonment, impulsivity, and self-harming behaviours may prompt individuals to seek professional help.

2. Seeking Professional Evaluation:

- Obtaining a diagnosis of BPD typically involves consulting mental health professionals, such as psychiatrists or psychologists, who specialise in diagnosing and treating personality disorders. These professionals conduct thorough assessments, which may include interviews, psychological evaluations, and discussions of medical history and symptoms.

3. Diagnostic Criteria:

- According to the Diagnostic and Statistical Manual of Mental Disorders (DSM-5), a diagnosis of borderline personality disorder is based on specific criteria, including patterns of unstable relationships, self-image disturbances, impulsivity, and marked mood instability. Professionals evaluate the presence and severity of these symptoms to determine if BPD criteria are met.

4. Relief and Validation:

- Receiving a formal diagnosis can bring a mix of emotions. For some, it provides a sense of relief—a validation of their experiences and struggles. It offers an explanation for the challenges they've faced, connecting dots that may have felt disconnected for years.

Acceptance and Moving Forward

1. Coming to Terms with the Diagnosis:

- Accepting a diagnosis of BPD can be a complex and deeply personal journey. It involves acknowledging and understanding the impact of the disorder on one's life, relationships, and sense of self. This process may involve grieving for the losses associated with BPD and recognising that the disorder does not define one's entire identity.

2. Education and Self-Awareness:

 - Education about BPD—its symptoms, causes, and treatment options—is instrumental in fostering self-awareness and empowerment. Learning about effective therapies, such as Dialectical Behaviour Therapy (DBT) or Cognitive Behavioural Therapy (CBT), can provide hope and practical strategies for managing symptoms and improving quality of life.

3. Building a Support Network:

  - Establishing a support network of understanding family members, friends, or support groups can be invaluable in the journey of acceptance. Sharing experiences with others who have BPD or loved ones who understand can provide emotional validation, encouragement, and practical guidance.

4. Embracing Personal Growth:

  - Acceptance of BPD can pave the way for personal growth and resilience. It involves developing coping skills, enhancing emotional regulation, and fostering healthier relationships. Through therapy and self-reflection, individuals can cultivate a stronger sense of self-worth and find meaning in their journey toward healing.

Diagnosis and acceptance of borderline personality disorder mark the beginning of a transformative journey —a journey of self-discovery, healing, and empowerment. By embracing the complexities of BPD with compassion and understanding, individuals can navigate challenges, build resilience, and ultimately thrive in their lives. Through education, support, and effective treatment, acceptance becomes a pivotal step toward reclaiming control and living authentically.

Coping with the initial diagnosis and coming to terms with living with BPD.

Receiving a diagnosis of borderline personality disorder (BPD) can be a profoundly challenging experience. It often marks the beginning of a journey filled with uncertainty, introspection, and emotional upheaval. Yet, amidst the whirlwind of emotions, there lies a path towards understanding, acceptance, and ultimately, finding ways to live a fulfilling life despite the challenges posed by BPD.

The Initial Impact

The moment you receive the diagnosis of BPD, it can feel like a seismic shift in your understanding of yourself and your life. For many, it may come as a relief, finally giving a name to the emotional turmoil and relational difficulties they've been experiencing. For others, it can be overwhelming, stirring up fears of stigma, self-doubt, and questions about what the future holds.

Processing Emotions

In the wake of diagnosis, a tidal wave of emotions is common. There may be grief for the perceived loss of a 'normal' life, anger at oneself or the circumstances, and fear of how others will perceive you. It's crucial to acknowledge and process these emotions without judgment. They are valid responses to a significant life event and denying them only prolongs the healing process.

Seeking Knowledge and Support

Understanding BPD is a critical step in coming to terms with it. Educating yourself about the disorder—its symptoms, causes, and treatment options—empowers you to make informed decisions about your health and well-being. This knowledge also helps counteract misconceptions and stigma, both internally and in your interactions with others.

Seeking support is equally vital. Whether from therapists specialising in BPD, support groups, or trusted friends and family members, having a network of understanding individuals can provide comfort, guidance, and a sense of belonging during difficult times.

Embracing Treatment and Recovery

Treatment for BPD often involves a multifaceted approach that may include therapy, medication, and lifestyle adjustments. Committing to treatment can be daunting, but it's a powerful step towards managing symptoms and improving overall quality of life. Therapy, especially dialectical behaviour therapy (DBT), has shown significant effectiveness in helping individuals with BPD regulate emotions, manage relationships, and build resilience.

Cultivating Self-Compassion

Living with BPD can be characterised by intense self-criticism and feelings of inadequacy. Practicing self-compassion—being kind and understanding towards oneself, especially in times of distress—is transformative. It involves treating yourself with the same empathy and care that you would offer to a loved one facing similar challenges.

Finding Meaning and Purpose

While BPD may present obstacles, it doesn't define your entire existence. Discovering and nurturing interests, hobbies, and relationships that bring joy and fulfilment can provide a sense of purpose beyond the diagnosis. Engaging in creative outlets, volunteering, or pursuing educational goals are ways to cultivate a meaningful life and strengthen resilience.

Embracing the Journey

Coming to terms with living with BPD is not a linear process; it's a journey marked by progress, setbacks, and moments of profound growth. There will be days when the weight feels unbearable and others when hope and resilience shine through. Each step, no matter how small, is a testament to your courage and determination to live authentically despite the challenges.

Ultimately, coping with the initial diagnosis of BPD and embracing life with the disorder involves a blend of self-awareness, self-compassion, and a commitment to seeking support and treatment. It's a journey that is uniquely yours, shaped by your experiences, strengths, and the relationships you cultivate along the way.

Remember, you are not alone in this journey. With time, patience, and the right support, it is possible to find stability, acceptance, and a fulfilling life beyond the diagnosis of borderline personality disorder.

Chapter 3.

Building a Support System

- The importance of supportive relationships and finding understanding.

Building a Support System

Receiving a diagnosis of borderline personality disorder (BPD) marks the beginning of a journey that often necessitates a robust support system. This network of understanding individuals—whether friends, family, therapists, or support groups—plays a pivotal role in providing comfort, guidance, and stability during times of emotional turmoil and personal growth.

Understanding Your Needs

Navigating life with BPD can be complex and emotionally taxing. Recognising your needs and identifying what kind of support would be most beneficial to you is a crucial first step. This may include emotional support, practical assistance with daily tasks, or someone to talk to during difficult moments. Each person's needs are unique, so take the time to reflect on what would be most helpful for you.

Seeking Professional Help

Therapy is often a cornerstone of treatment for BPD, and finding a therapist who specialises in the disorder can provide invaluable support. Dialectical Behaviour Therapy (DBT) is particularly effective for individuals with BPD, focusing on skills such as mindfulness, emotion regulation, interpersonal effectiveness, and distress tolerance. A therapist can offer guidance, validation, and tools to help you manage symptoms and improve your quality of life.

Educating Your Support System

Many people are unfamiliar with BPD and may have misconceptions about the disorder. Educating your support system—whether it's friends, family members, or colleagues—can help foster understanding, empathy, and effective communication. Share reliable resources, such as articles or books, and encourage open dialogue about your experiences, challenges, and goals. This mutual understanding can strengthen relationships and create a more supportive environment.

Connecting with Peers

Joining a support group specifically for individuals with BPD can provide a sense of community and validation. Interacting with peers who share similar experiences can reduce feelings of isolation and offer practical insights into coping strategies that have worked for others. Online forums, local support groups, or structured therapy groups led by trained professionals are options to explore based on your comfort level and preferences.

Building Trust and Communication

Effective communication is essential in any support system. Clearly expressing your needs, boundaries, and preferences allows others to provide meaningful support without overstepping. Building trust within your support network involves being open about your feelings and experiences while also respecting the perspectives and boundaries of others. Trust grows through consistent, empathetic communication and mutual respect.

Diversifying Your Support

A diverse support system includes different types of relationships and resources that cater to various aspects of your life. While friends and family offer emotional support, professionals such as therapists provide specialised guidance and treatment. Engaging in hobbies, joining community activities, or exploring spiritual or religious practices can also enrich your support network by connecting you with like-minded individuals who share common interests and values.

Taking Care of Yourself

Self-care is foundational to maintaining a healthy support system. Prioritise activities that promote physical, emotional, and mental well-being, such as exercise, adequate sleep, healthy eating, and relaxation techniques like meditation or yoga. Taking care of yourself not only enhances your ability to cope with BPD symptoms but also strengthens your capacity to engage meaningfully with your support system.

Adapting and Evolving

As you navigate life with BPD, your needs and preferences may change over time. Be open to reassessing and adjusting your support system accordingly. Some relationships may naturally evolve or fade, while new connections may emerge that better align with your current circumstances and goals. Embrace the process of growth and adaptation, recognising that building a supportive network is a dynamic and ongoing journey.

Finding Hope and Strength

Building a support system after being diagnosed with BPD is a courageous and empowering step towards managing the challenges of the disorder and fostering a fulfilling life. Surrounding yourself with understanding individuals who offer compassion, encouragement, and practical assistance can provide the strength and resilience needed to navigate the ups and downs of life with BPD.

Remember, you are not defined by your diagnosis. With the right support and self-care, it is possible to cultivate a meaningful and rewarding life that embraces both challenges and triumphs along the way.

The importance of supportive relationships and finding understanding

Receiving a diagnosis of borderline personality disorder (BPD) can be a deeply emotional and transformative experience. It often brings a mix of relief, validation, and uncertainty about the future. In this journey of self-discovery and growth, the role of supportive relationships and finding understanding from others cannot be overstated. These connections play a vital role in providing comfort, validation, and guidance, helping individuals navigate the complexities of living with BPD with greater resilience and hope.

Validation and Empathy

One of the most profound needs after a diagnosis of BPD is validation—being understood and acknowledged for one's experiences and emotions without judgment. Supportive relationships offer a safe space where individuals can express themselves openly, knowing that their feelings are recognised and accepted. This validation validates their struggles and challenges, validating their struggles and challenges, and is a crucial step towards healing.

Reducing Stigma and Misconceptions

BPD is often misunderstood and stigmatised, both within society and sometimes even within one's social circles. Supportive relationships play a crucial role in challenging these misconceptions and reducing stigma. When friends, family members, or colleagues take the time to educate themselves about BPD, they can offer more empathetic support, fostering an environment where individuals feel empowered to seek help and engage in treatment without fear of judgment.

Providing Practical Support

Living with BPD can present daily challenges, from managing intense emotions to navigating interpersonal relationships. Supportive relationships can offer practical assistance, such as helping with daily tasks during periods of emotional distress, accompanying to therapy appointments, or simply being a listening ear during difficult moments. These acts of support not only alleviate immediate stress but also demonstrate care and commitment to the well-being of the individual with BPD.

Building Trust and Stability

Trust is foundational in any relationship, and for individuals with BPD, building trust can be particularly significant. Supportive relationships foster a sense of security and stability, providing a reliable anchor during times of emotional turbulence. When individuals feel trusted and supported, they are more likely to engage openly in therapy, follow treatment plans, and develop healthier coping mechanisms—all of which contribute to long-term stability and well-being.

Encouraging Growth and Recovery

Recovery from BPD is a journey that often involves personal growth, self-awareness, and learning new skills to manage symptoms effectively. Supportive relationships play a pivotal role in this process by encouraging individuals to explore their strengths, face challenges with resilience, and celebrate their progress, no matter how small. By offering encouragement and constructive feedback, supportive allies become catalysts for growth and recovery.

Finding Understanding and Connection

At its core, finding understanding after a diagnosis of BPD is about fostering genuine connections based on empathy, compassion, and mutual respect. Supportive relationships provide a sense of belonging and solidarity, reminding individuals that they are not alone in their journey. Whether through shared experiences, thoughtful conversations, or moments of laughter and joy, these connections enrich life and reinforce the belief that healing and hope are attainable.

The Power of Compassion

Above all, supportive relationships embody the power of compassion—the ability to see beyond symptoms and diagnoses to recognise the inherent worth and dignity of every individual. By embracing compassion, both within oneself and in relationships, individuals with BPD can cultivate a sense of self-acceptance and build fulfilling connections that contribute to their overall well-being.

Embracing a Journey of Healing

Navigating life with BPD is a deeply personal and transformative journey, shaped by the support and understanding of those who walk alongside. Each relationship—whether with friends, family, therapists, or peers—contributes to a tapestry of resilience, hope, and healing. By nurturing supportive relationships and finding understanding after a diagnosis of BPD, individuals can embrace the journey towards a more fulfilling and empowered life, where compassion and connection pave the way to brighter horizons.

Remember, you deserve understanding and support as you navigate the challenges and celebrate the victories of living with BPD. Together, we can create a world where empathy and acceptance flourish, offering hope and healing to all.

Chapter 4.

Cognitive Behavioural Strategies

- Practical techniques for managing intense emotions and impulsivity.

Cognitive Behavioural Strategies

Borderline Personality Disorder (BPD) is characterised by intense emotional experiences, unstable relationships, and a fluctuating sense of self. While living with BPD can be challenging, cognitive-behavioural strategies offer effective tools to help manage symptoms, improve emotional regulation, and enhance overall quality of life. By incorporating these strategies into daily life, individuals with BPD can develop healthier thinking patterns and behaviours, fostering greater emotional stability and well-being.

1. Understanding Cognitive-Behavioural Therapy (CBT)

Cognitive-Behavioural Therapy (CBT) is a widely recognised therapeutic approach that focuses on identifying and changing negative thought patterns and behaviours. For individuals with BPD, CBT can be particularly beneficial in addressing distorted thinking, improving emotional regulation, and developing healthier coping mechanisms. The core principles of CBT involve recognising the connection between thoughts, emotions, and behaviours, and making conscious efforts to alter them for better outcomes.

2. Identifying and Challenging Negative Thoughts

A fundamental aspect of CBT is recognising and challenging negative thought patterns. Individuals with BPD often experience distorted thinking, such as black-and-white thinking, catastrophising, or overgeneralizing. By identifying these patterns, individuals can begin to question their validity and replace them with more balanced and realistic thoughts.

Steps to Challenge Negative Thoughts:

- Identify the Negative Thought: Pay attention to automatic negative thoughts that arise in response to specific situations.

- Examine the Evidence: Assess the evidence supporting and contradicting the negative thought.

- Consider Alternative Perspectives: Explore other ways to interpret the situation that are less extreme and more balanced.

- Replace the Thought: Replace the negative thought with a more rational and constructive one.

3. Practicing Mindfulness and Distress Tolerance

Mindfulness involves being present in the moment without judgment. For individuals with BPD, mindfulness can help reduce emotional reactivity and increase awareness of thoughts and feelings. Distress tolerance skills, a key component of Dialectical Behaviour Therapy (DBT), can also be integrated into a CBT framework to help manage intense emotions without resorting to self-destructive behaviours.

Mindfulness Practices:

- Breathing Exercises: Focus on your breath, inhaling deeply and exhaling slowly to ground yourself in the present moment.

- Body Scan: Pay attention to physical sensations in your body, moving your focus from head to toe.

- Mindful Observation: Engage your senses by observing your surroundings with curiosity and without judgment.

Distress Tolerance Skills:

- Self-Soothing: Engage in activities that provide comfort, such as listening to soothing music, taking a warm bath, or practicing gentle yoga.

- Distraction: Redirect your attention to activities that divert your focus from distressing thoughts, such as reading, drawing, or engaging in a hobby.

- Crisis Survival Strategies: Use techniques like cold-water immersion (splashing your face with cold water) to rapidly decrease emotional intensity.

4. Emotion Regulation Techniques

Emotion regulation is crucial for individuals with BPD who often experience intense and rapidly changing emotions. CBT offers strategies to help individuals recognise, understand, and manage their emotions more effectively.

Emotion Regulation Strategies:

- Labelling Emotions: Identify and name the emotions you are experiencing to gain clarity and perspective.

- Opposite Action: Engage in behaviours opposite to what your emotions urge you to do (e.g., if feeling angry, try engaging in a calming activity).

- Problem-Solving: Address the root cause of distressing emotions by developing practical solutions to problems.

5. Interpersonal Effectiveness Skills

BPD can significantly impact relationships, leading to conflicts and instability. CBT includes interpersonal effectiveness skills to help individuals communicate more effectively, set healthy boundaries, and maintain stable relationships.

Interpersonal Effectiveness Skills:

- Assertiveness Training: Learn to express your needs, desires, and boundaries clearly and respectfully.

- Active Listening: Practice attentive listening to understand others' perspectives and validate their feelings.

- Negotiation: Develop skills to negotiate and find mutually beneficial solutions in conflicts.

6. Building a Support Network

Incorporating cognitive-behavioural strategies into daily life can be challenging, especially without support. Building a network of understanding individuals, including therapists, support groups, friends, and family, can provide the encouragement and reinforcement needed to stay committed to these strategies.

Cognitive-behavioural strategies offer practical and effective tools for managing the complexities of borderline personality disorder. By identifying and challenging negative thoughts, practicing mindfulness and distress tolerance, regulating emotions, and enhancing interpersonal skills, individuals with BPD can gain greater control over their lives and foster healthier relationships. Remember, progress takes time and effort, but with persistence and support, it is possible to achieve a more stable and fulfilling life.

Practical techniques for managing intense emotions and impulsivity.

Living with Borderline Personality Disorder (BPD) often means navigating a landscape of intense emotions and impulsive behaviours. These experiences can be overwhelming and challenging, but practical techniques can provide tools to manage these symptoms effectively. By incorporating these strategies into daily life, individuals with BPD can cultivate greater emotional stability and control over impulsive actions, fostering a more balanced and fulfilling life.

1. Grounding Techniques for Emotional Intensity

Grounding techniques help bring focus to the present moment, providing a sense of stability and calm during emotional upheaval. These techniques can interrupt the cycle of intense emotions and offer a way to regain control.

Grounding Techniques:

- 5-4-3-2-1 Technique: Identify five things you can see, four things you can touch, three things you can hear, two things you can smell, and one thing you can taste. This sensory exercise helps anchor you in the present.

- Deep Breathing: Inhale deeply for a count of four, hold for four, and exhale for four. Repeat several times to calm the nervous system and reduce emotional intensity.

- Physical Grounding: Hold an ice cube, run your hands under cold water, or stomp your feet. These physical sensations can divert your focus from intense emotions.

2. Mindfulness Practices for Emotional Regulation

Mindfulness involves paying attention to the present moment with a non-judgmental attitude. Regular mindfulness practice can help increase awareness of emotions and reduce reactivity.

Mindfulness Practices:

- Body Scan Meditation: Slowly scan your body from head to toe, noting any areas of tension or discomfort. This practice helps you become more aware of your physical and emotional state.

- Breath Awareness: Focus on your breath, noticing the sensation of air entering and leaving your body. When your mind wanders, gently bring your attention back to your breath.

- Mindful Observation: Observe your surroundings without judgment. Notice the colours, shapes, and textures around you, fully engaging your senses.

3. Distress Tolerance Skills for Crisis Moments

Distress tolerance skills are designed to help you survive immediate emotional crises without making the situation worse. These techniques provide temporary relief and a way to endure distressing moments.

Distress Tolerance Skills:

- TIPP (Temperature, Intense Exercise, Paced Breathing, Progressive Relaxation):

  - Temperature: Change your body temperature quickly by holding ice, splashing your face with cold water, or taking a cold shower.

  - Intense Exercise: Engage in vigorous physical activity to burn off excess emotional energy.

  - Paced Breathing: Slow your breathing with deep, deliberate breaths to calm your nervous system.

  - Progressive Relaxation: Tense and relax different muscle groups in your body to release physical tension.

- Self-Soothing: Use your senses to comfort yourself. Light a scented candle, listen to calming music, wrap yourself in a soft blanket, or enjoy a favourite treat.

- Distraction: Redirect your attention to something engaging, such as a hobby, a book, a movie, or a puzzle.

4. Cognitive Restructuring for Impulsive Thoughts

Cognitive restructuring involves identifying and challenging distorted or irrational thoughts that can lead to impulsive behaviours. By reshaping these thoughts, you can reduce impulsivity and make more considered decisions.

Steps for Cognitive Restructuring:

Identify the Thought: Recognise the impulsive or negative thought that arises in response to a situation.

- Challenge the Thought: Ask yourself if the thought is based on facts or assumptions. Look for evidence that supports or contradicts it.

- Reframe the Thought: Replace the impulsive thought with a more balanced and rational perspective. For example, change "I must react now" to "I can take a moment to think before I act."

5. Behavioural Techniques for Managing Impulsivity

Behavioural techniques help modify actions and create new, healthier habits. These strategies can reduce impulsive behaviours and increase self-control.

Behavioural Techniques:

- Delay Technique: When you feel the urge to act impulsively, delay the action for a set period, such as 10 minutes. Use this time to consider the potential consequences and alternatives.

- Pros and Cons List: Make a list of the pros and cons of impulsive behaviour. Reviewing this list can help you make more informed decisions.

- Pre-commitment: Create a plan or commitment in advance to avoid impulsive actions. For example, if you tend to overspend, set a budget and stick to it or leave your credit cards at home.

6. Building a Supportive Environment

Creating a supportive environment can enhance your ability to manage intense emotions and impulsivity. Surround yourself with understanding individuals who respect your boundaries and offer encouragement.

Supportive Environment Tips:

- Communicate Your Needs: Clearly express your needs and boundaries to those around you. Let them know how they can support you during difficult times.

- Seek Professional Help: Work with a therapist who specialises in BPD to develop personalised strategies and receive guidance.

- Join Support Groups: Connect with others who have similar experiences. Support groups offer a sense of community and shared understanding.

Managing intense emotions and impulsivity in borderline personality disorder is challenging, but practical techniques can provide effective tools to navigate these experiences. By incorporating grounding techniques, mindfulness practices, distress tolerance skills, cognitive restructuring, behavioural strategies, and building a supportive environment, individuals with BPD can gain greater control over their emotions and actions. Remember, progress takes time and effort, but with persistence and support, it is possible to achieve a more balanced and fulfilling life.

Chapter 5.

Dialectical Behaviour Therapy

- Explanation of DBT principles and how they can be applied in daily life.

Dialectical Behaviour Therapy

Borderline Personality Disorder (BPD) is a complex mental health condition characterised by intense emotions, unstable relationships, and impulsive behaviours. For many individuals with BPD, these symptoms can be overwhelming and difficult to manage. Dialectical Behaviour Therapy (DBT), developed by psychologist Marsha M. Linehan, has emerged as one of the most effective treatments for BPD. This therapeutic approach blends cognitive-behavioural techniques with mindfulness practices, offering a structured and supportive framework for individuals seeking to improve their emotional regulation, interpersonal skills, and overall quality of life.

The Foundation of DBT

DBT is rooted in the concept of "dialectics," which involves understanding and integrating opposing perspectives. The central dialectic in DBT is the balance between acceptance and change—accepting oneself and one's experiences while simultaneously working towards positive change. This dual focus helps individuals with BPD cultivate self-compassion while developing practical skills to manage their symptoms.

Core Components of DBT

DBT comprises four main components, each addressing different aspects of emotional and behavioural regulation:

1. Mindfulness: Cultivating Present-Moment Awareness

Mindfulness is the practice of being fully present and engaged in the current moment without judgment. For individuals with BPD, mindfulness helps increase awareness of thoughts, emotions, and physical sensations, allowing for greater emotional regulation and a reduction in impulsive reactions.

Mindfulness Practices:

- Observing: Notice and describe what you are experiencing internally and externally.

- Describing: Put words to your experiences, labelling thoughts and feelings without judgment.

- Participating: Fully engage in the present activity, letting go of distractions and self-criticism.

2. Emotion Regulation: Managing Intense Emotions

Emotion regulation skills help individuals with BPD understand and manage their intense emotional responses. These techniques aim to reduce vulnerability to negative emotions and increase positive emotional experiences.

Emotion Regulation Skills:

- Identifying Emotions: Learn to recognise and label your emotions accurately.

- Reducing Vulnerability: Take care of your physical and mental health through regular exercise, balanced nutrition, adequate sleep, and stress management.

- Building Positive Experiences: Engage in activities that bring joy and satisfaction to create a buffer against negative emotions.

3. Distress Tolerance: Surviving Crisis Moments

Distress tolerance skills provide tools to endure and cope with emotional crises without resorting to self-destructive behaviours. These techniques offer immediate relief and help individuals navigate distressing situations safely.

Distress Tolerance Skills:

- TIPP (Temperature, Intense Exercise, Paced Breathing, Progressive Relaxation): Techniques to quickly reduce emotional arousal.

- Self-Soothing: Use your senses to comfort yourself through calming activities.

- Distraction: Redirect your focus to engaging activities that temporarily take your mind off the distress.

4. Interpersonal Effectiveness: Navigating Relationships

Interpersonal effectiveness skills teach individuals with BPD how to communicate more effectively, set healthy boundaries, and maintain stable relationships. These skills are crucial for managing the interpersonal conflicts that often arise in BPD.

Interpersonal Effectiveness Skills:

- DEAR MAN (Describe, Express, Assert, Reinforce, Mindful, Appear Confident, Negotiate): A framework for effective communication.

- GIVE (Gentle, Interested, Validate, Easy Manner): Strategies for maintaining positive relationships.

- FAST (Fair, Apologies, Stick to Values, Truthful): Guidelines for maintaining self-respect in interactions.

The Structure of DBT

DBT is typically delivered in three main formats:

1. Individual Therapy:

Weekly one-on-one sessions with a trained DBT therapist focus on addressing personal challenges and applying DBT skills to real-life situations. Therapists provide support, guidance, and validation, helping clients navigate their unique experiences with BPD.

2. Skills Training Groups:

Weekly group sessions focus on teaching and practicing DBT skills in a supportive environment. These groups provide an opportunity to learn from others' experiences and to receive feedback and encouragement.

3. Phone Coaching:

Between sessions, clients have access to phone coaching, where they can seek immediate support from their therapist during crises or when they need help applying DBT skills in real-time.

The Benefits of DBT

Research has shown that DBT is highly effective in reducing the symptoms of BPD. Benefits include:

- Decreased frequency and severity of self-harming behaviours and suicidal ideation.

- Improved emotional regulation and reduction in emotional outbursts.

- Enhanced interpersonal relationships and communication skills.

- Increased ability to tolerate distress and manage crises.

- Greater overall quality of life and well-being.

Dialectical Behaviour Therapy offers a comprehensive and compassionate approach to managing borderline personality disorder. By blending acceptance and change, DBT equips individuals with the skills needed to navigate intense emotions, build healthier relationships, and create a more balanced and fulfilling life. While the journey with BPD can be challenging, DBT provides a structured path towards healing and empowerment, fostering resilience and hope along the way.

Explanation of DBT principles and how they can be applied in daily life.

Borderline Personality Disorder (BPD) is marked by intense emotions, unstable relationships, and impulsive behaviours, making daily life often feel unpredictable and overwhelming. Dialectical Behaviour Therapy (DBT), developed by psychologist Marsha M. Linehan, provides a structured approach to help individuals manage these challenges. DBT combines cognitive-behavioural techniques with mindfulness practices, focusing on skills for emotional regulation, distress tolerance, interpersonal effectiveness, and mindfulness. Understanding and applying DBT principles can significantly enhance the quality of life for individuals with BPD.

Core Principles of DBT

1. Mindfulness: Cultivating Present-Moment Awareness

- Principle: Mindfulness involves being fully present and aware in the current moment without judgment.

- Application in Daily Life: Practice mindfulness by engaging in activities with full attention. For instance, when eating, focus on the taste, texture, and aroma of the food. During conversations, listen actively without planning your response. Use mindfulness exercises, such as deep breathing or body scans, to centre yourself when feeling overwhelmed.

2. Emotion Regulation: Managing Intense Emotions

- Principle: Emotion regulation skills help individuals understand and manage their emotional responses effectively.

- Application in Daily Life: Start by identifying and labelling your emotions throughout the day. Keep a journal to track what triggers intense emotions and note how you respond. Engage in activities that promote positive emotions, such as hobbies, exercise, or spending time with loved ones. Develop a self-care routine that includes regular sleep, balanced nutrition, and stress management practices.

3. Distress Tolerance: Surviving Crisis Moments

- Principle: Distress tolerance skills provide tools to endure and cope with emotional crises without resorting to harmful behaviours.

- Application in Daily Life: Use the TIPP (Temperature, Intense Exercise, Paced Breathing, Progressive Relaxation) skills when experiencing intense distress. For example, splash your face with cold water or hold an ice cube to quickly change your body's physical response. Engage in intense physical activity like running or dancing to release pent-up energy. Practice paced breathing by inhaling deeply for a count of four, holding for four, and exhaling for four.

4. Interpersonal Effectiveness: Navigating Relationships

   - Principle: Interpersonal effectiveness skills help individuals communicate, set healthy boundaries, and maintain stable relationships.

   - Application in Daily Life: Use the DEAR MAN (Describe, Express, Assert, Reinforce, Mindful, Appear Confident, Negotiate) technique for effective communication. For instance, when asking for something from a friend, clearly describe what you need, express your feelings, assert your request, and reinforce the benefits. Practice active listening and validation in conversations to build rapport and trust. Set boundaries by clearly stating your limits and sticking to them, even when it feels uncomfortable.

Practical Examples of Applying DBT Skills

1. Mindfulness in Daily Routines:

   - Morning Routine: Start your day with a brief mindfulness exercise, such as a 5-minute breathing meditation or mindful stretching. This sets a calm tone for the day.

- Commute: Use your commute to practice mindfulness by observing your surroundings, noticing your breath, or listening to a guided meditation.

2. Emotion Regulation Techniques:

- Identifying Triggers: Keep a diary to note situations that trigger strong emotional reactions. Over time, this helps in identifying patterns and preparing for similar situations in the future.

- Positive Activities: Schedule regular activities that bring joy and relaxation, such as reading, gardening, or engaging in creative pursuits. These activities can buffer against negative emotions.

3. Distress Tolerance in Action:

- Crisis Kit: Create a crisis kit with items that help you cope during distressing times, such as stress balls, soothing music, scented candles, or comforting photographs.

- Distraction Techniques: When overwhelmed, use distraction techniques like watching a favourite TV show, doing a puzzle, or engaging in a hobby that fully absorbs your attention.

4. Interpersonal Effectiveness at Work:

- Assertive Communication: In a work setting, use DEAR MAN to request a change in your schedule. Describe your current workload, express how it affects you, assert your request for adjustments, and reinforce how this change benefits the team.

- Setting Boundaries: If a colleague frequently interrupts you, politely but firmly set a boundary by saying, "I appreciate your input, but I need uninterrupted time to complete this task. Can we discuss this later?"

Dialectical Behaviour Therapy offers a comprehensive framework for managing the complexities of borderline personality disorder. By incorporating DBT principles into daily life, individuals with BPD can develop greater emotional resilience, improve their relationships, and navigate challenges with more confidence and stability. The journey with BPD is undoubtedly challenging, but with the right tools and support, it is possible to lead a more balanced and fulfilling life. Remember, progress takes time and practice, so be patient and compassionate with yourself as you integrate these skills into your daily routine.

Chapter 6.

Mindfulness and Grounding Techniques

- Exercises to stay present and manage dissociation.

Mindfulness and Grounding Techniques

Borderline Personality Disorder (BPD) is characterised by intense emotional experiences, unstable relationships, and impulsive behaviours, often leaving individuals feeling overwhelmed and disconnected. Mindfulness and grounding techniques offer practical tools to help manage these symptoms by promoting present-moment awareness and providing a sense of stability. By incorporating these practices into daily life, individuals with BPD can enhance emotional regulation, reduce distress, and foster a greater sense of well-being.

Understanding Mindfulness

Mindfulness involves paying attention to the present moment with curiosity and without judgment. This practice helps individuals become more aware of their thoughts, feelings, and physical sensations, allowing them to respond to situations with greater clarity and calmness. For those with BPD, mindfulness can reduce emotional reactivity and improve self-awareness, providing a solid foundation for managing the disorder.

Mindfulness Practices for Daily Life

1. Breath Awareness:

  - Technique: Sit or lie down comfortably. Focus on your breath as it enters and leaves your body. Notice the rise and fall of your chest and abdomen. If your mind wanders, gently bring your attention back to your breath.

  - Application: Use breath awareness during moments of stress or anxiety to ground yourself and regain composure.

2. Body Scan:

  - Technique: Close your eyes and bring your attention to different parts of your body, starting from your toes and moving up to your head. Notice any sensations, tension, or discomfort without trying to change anything.

  - Application: Practice the body scan before bed to relax and prepare for sleep, or during the day to reconnect with your physical self.

3. Mindful Eating:

- Technique: Eat a meal or snack slowly, paying full attention to the taste, texture, smell, and appearance of the food. Notice the sensations in your mouth and body as you eat.

- Application: Use mindful eating to enhance your enjoyment of food and to cultivate a mindful attitude in everyday activities.

4. Mindful Walking:

- Technique: Walk slowly and deliberately, focusing on the sensation of your feet touching the ground and the movement of your legs. Notice the sights, sounds, and smells around you.

- Application: Incorporate mindful walking into your daily routine, such as during your commute or when walking the dog, to foster a sense of calm and presence.

Grounding Techniques for Emotional Stability

Grounding techniques help individuals stay connected to the present moment, particularly during times of distress or emotional intensity. These techniques provide a sense of safety and stability, making it easier to manage overwhelming emotions and impulses.

1. 5-4-3-2-1 Technique:

   - Technique: Identify five things you can see, four things you can touch, three things you can hear, two things you can smell, and one thing you can taste. Engage your senses fully in the process.

   - Application: Use this technique when you feel disconnected or overwhelmed to anchor yourself in the present moment.

2. Physical Grounding:

- Technique: Hold an ice cube, splash your face with cold water, or touch a textured object. Focus on the physical sensations these actions create.

- Application: Use physical grounding techniques during intense emotional episodes to redirect your focus and calm your nervous system.

3. Progressive Muscle Relaxation:

- Technique: Tense and then relax different muscle groups in your body, starting from your toes and moving up to your head. Notice the difference between tension and relaxation.

- Application: Practice progressive muscle relaxation when you feel anxious or tense to release physical and emotional stress.

4. Visualisation:

- Technique: Close your eyes and imagine a safe, calming place. It could be a beach, forest, or a favourite room. Engage all your senses to make the visualisation as vivid as possible.

- Application: Use visualisation during moments of high stress or when you need a mental break to create a sense of peace and safety.

Incorporating Mindfulness and Grounding into Daily Life

Integrating mindfulness and grounding techniques into your daily routine can enhance their effectiveness and make them a natural part of your coping strategy. Here are some tips to help you incorporate these practices:

1. Create a Routine:

   - Set aside specific times each day for mindfulness and grounding exercises, such as first thing in the morning, during lunch breaks, or before bed.

2. Start Small:

   - Begin with short, manageable sessions (5-10 minutes) and gradually increase the duration as you become more comfortable with the practices.

3. Use Reminders:

   - Set reminders on your phone or place sticky notes around your living space to prompt you to practice mindfulness and grounding throughout the day.

4. Combine with Daily Activities:

   - Integrate mindfulness into everyday tasks like brushing your teeth, washing dishes, or commuting to work to make these practices more seamless and sustainable.

5. Seek Support:

   - Join mindfulness or meditation groups, or work with a therapist trained in mindfulness-based therapies to receive guidance and encouragement.

Mindfulness and grounding techniques are powerful tools for managing the intense emotions and impulsivity associated with borderline personality disorder. By fostering present-moment awareness and providing a sense of stability, these practices can significantly enhance emotional regulation and overall well-being. With consistent practice and integration into daily life, individuals with BPD can cultivate a greater sense of control and resilience, making it easier to navigate the challenges of the disorder. Remember, the journey to emotional stability and well-being is ongoing, and every step taken towards mindfulness and grounding is a step towards a more balanced and fulfilling life.

Exercises to stay present and manage dissociation

Borderline Personality Disorder (BPD) can often involve periods of dissociation, where individuals feel disconnected from their thoughts, feelings, or surroundings. This can be distressing and disorienting, making it challenging to stay present and grounded. However, there are several exercises that can help manage dissociation and promote a sense of presence. These practices can provide stability and enhance overall well-being for individuals with BPD.

Understanding Dissociation in BPD

Dissociation is a mental process where a person disconnects from their thoughts, feelings, memories, or sense of identity. For those with BPD, dissociation can occur as a coping mechanism in response to stress, trauma, or overwhelming emotions. It may manifest as feeling detached from reality, experiencing gaps in memory, or feeling as if the world around them is unreal. While dissociation is a way to protect oneself from emotional pain, it can also hinder daily functioning and relationships.

Exercises to Stay Present and Manage Dissociation

1. Grounding Techniques

Grounding techniques are practical exercises that help anchor individuals in the present moment. These techniques engage the senses and create a connection to the here and now, counteracting the effects of dissociation.

- 5-4-3-2-1 Exercise:

    - Identify five things you can see around you.

    - Identify four things you can touch.

    - Identify three things you can hear.

    - Identify two things you can smell.

    - Identify one thing you can taste.

- Application: This exercise can be used anytime you start to feel disconnected or overwhelmed. It helps to quickly bring your attention back to the present moment by engaging your senses.

- Physical Grounding:

- Hold an ice cube in your hand and focus on the sensation of cold.

- Run your hands under cold water.

- Stomp your feet on the ground or walk barefoot on a textured surface.

- Application: Physical grounding is effective during intense moments of dissociation. The strong sensory input helps to anchor your awareness in your body.

2. Mindfulness Practices

Mindfulness involves paying attention to the present moment without judgment. Regular mindfulness practice can help reduce the frequency and intensity of dissociation by increasing awareness and promoting a sense of calm.

- Breath Awareness:

    - Sit comfortably and close your eyes.

    - Focus on your breath as it enters and leaves your body.

    - Notice the sensation of the breath in your nostrils, chest, and abdomen.

    - If your mind wanders, gently bring your focus back to your breath.

    - Application: Practice breath awareness daily for a few minutes. This exercise helps create a habit of returning to the present moment.

- Body Scan Meditation:

  - Lie down or sit comfortably and close your eyes.

  - Bring your attention to different parts of your body, starting from your toes and moving up to your head.

  - Notice any sensations, tension, or discomfort in each area without trying to change anything.

  - Application: Use the body scan meditation before bed or during breaks to reconnect with your body and reduce dissociative symptoms.

3. Sensory Engagement

Engaging the senses can help counteract dissociation by providing strong, immediate stimuli that draw attention back to the present moment.

- Sensory Kits:

  - Create a kit with items that engage your senses, such as scented candles, textured objects, or flavoured lozenges.

  - Use these items when you start to feel disconnected.

  - Application: Keep the sensory kit accessible, such as in your bag or at your desk, so you can use it whenever you need to ground yourself.

- Mindful Eating:

  - Eat a small piece of food, such as a raisin or a piece of chocolate, slowly and mindfully.

  - Notice the texture, taste, and aroma of the food.

  - Pay attention to the sensation of chewing and swallowing.

  - Application: Use mindful eating during meals or snacks to practice staying present and engaged with your senses.

4. Visualisation Techniques

Visualisation exercises can help create a mental anchor that promotes a sense of safety and presence.

- Safe Place Visualization:

  - Close your eyes and imagine a place where you feel completely safe and relaxed.

  - It could be a real place or a fictional one.

  - Engage all your senses to make the visualisation vivid—notice the colours, sounds, smells, and textures.

 - Application: Use this visualisation during stressful times to create a mental escape and reduce dissociative feelings.

- Guided Imagery:

  - Listen to a guided imagery recording that leads you through a calming scenario, such as walking through a forest or lying on a beach.

- Focus on the imagery and allow yourself to fully immerse in the experience.

- Application Guided imagery recordings are available online or through meditation apps. Use them during moments of stress or before bed to promote relaxation and presence.

5. Cognitive Techniques

Cognitive techniques involve using thought processes to stay connected to reality and the present moment.

- Reality Testing:

- Ask yourself questions to determine whether your perceptions match reality, such as "What is the date and time?" or "Where am I right now?"

- Application: Use reality testing when you start to feel detached or unsure about what is real. It helps reinforce your connection to the present moment.

- Positive Affirmations:

  - Create a list of positive affirmations or grounding statements, such as "I am here and now" or "I am safe."

  - Repeat these affirmations to yourself during moments of dissociation.

  - Application: Write your affirmations on sticky notes and place them in visible locations, such as on your mirror or computer, to remind yourself of them regularly.

Managing dissociation in borderline personality disorder requires consistent practice and a variety of techniques. Grounding exercises, mindfulness practices, sensory engagement, visualisation techniques, and cognitive strategies can all play a role in helping individuals stay present and connected to the here and now. By incorporating these exercises into daily life, those with BPD can reduce the impact of dissociation, enhance their emotional stability, and improve their overall quality of life. Remember, progress takes time and effort, so be patient with yourself as you explore and integrate these practices.

Chapter 7.

Navigating Relationships

- How BPD affects relationships and strategies for healthier interactions.

Navigating Relationships

Borderline Personality Disorder (BPD) is characterised by intense emotions, fear of abandonment, and difficulties in maintaining stable relationships. These challenges can make navigating relationships particularly complex and stressful. However, with understanding and the right strategies, individuals with BPD can build and maintain healthy, fulfilling relationships. Here are some key approaches to managing relationships while living with BPD.

Understanding Relationship Challenges in BPD

Individuals with BPD often experience relationships as tumultuous and intense. Common relationship challenges include:

- Fear of Abandonment: Individuals with BPD may have an intense fear of being abandoned or rejected, leading to clingy or overly dependent behaviour.

- Emotional Instability: Rapid mood swings and intense emotional reactions can strain relationships and create misunderstandings.

- Black-and-White Thinking: Seeing people as all good or all bad, also known as splitting, can lead to volatile relationships.

- Impulsivity: Impulsive actions or decisions can harm relationships and create instability.

- Self-Image Issues: Inconsistent or unstable self-image can affect how individuals interact with others and perceive their relationships.

Strategies for Navigating Relationships

1. Develop Self-Awareness

   - Practice Mindfulness: Engage in mindfulness exercises to become more aware of your thoughts, emotions, and reactions. This awareness can help you identify triggers and patterns in your behaviour that affect relationships.

- Reflect on Past Relationships: Analyse past relationships to understand what worked and what didn't. Identify recurring issues and think about how you might address them differently in future relationships.

2. Communicate Effectively

- Use "I" Statements: Express your feelings and needs using "I" statements, such as "I feel upset when..." or "I need some time to process this." This approach reduces defensiveness and fosters open communication.

- Active Listening: Practice active listening by fully focusing on what the other person is saying without planning your response. Reflect back what you've heard to ensure understanding.

- Be Honest: Share your experiences and struggles with BPD openly with trusted individuals. Honesty builds trust and allows others to understand your perspective better.

3. Set Healthy Boundaries

- Know Your Limits: Understand your own emotional and physical limits and communicate them clearly to others. Boundaries help protect your well-being and prevent burnout.

- Assertiveness: Practice assertive communication to express your needs and boundaries without aggression. Use techniques like DEAR MAN (Describe, Express, Assert, Reinforce, Mindful, Appear Confident, Negotiate) to maintain healthy interactions.

4. Manage Emotional Reactions

- Emotion Regulation Skills: Use DBT (Dialectical Behaviour Therapy) skills, such as emotion regulation techniques, to manage intense emotions. Techniques like deep breathing, progressive muscle relaxation, and grounding exercises can help.

- Delay Reacting: When you feel a strong emotional reaction, take a moment to pause before responding. This delay can prevent impulsive reactions and allow for more thoughtful communication.

5. Seek Support

- Therapy: Engage in individual or group therapy to work on relationship skills and emotional regulation. Therapists can provide guidance and strategies tailored to your needs.

- Support Groups: Join support groups for individuals with BPD or those dealing with similar relationship challenges. Sharing experiences and strategies with others can be empowering and validating.

6. Build Trust Gradually

- Take Small Steps: Build trust in relationships gradually. Start with small acts of trust and gradually increase as the relationship strengthens.

- Consistency: Be consistent in your actions and communication. Consistency helps build reliability and trustworthiness in relationships.

7. Focus on Self-Care

- Prioritise Well-Being: Ensure you are taking care of your own physical and emotional health. Engage in regular self-care activities that promote relaxation and well-being.

- Balance: Maintain a balance between focusing on your needs and the needs of the relationship. Healthy relationships thrive on mutual respect and care.

Navigating relationships with borderline personality disorder can be challenging, but it is possible to build and maintain healthy, fulfilling connections with the right strategies and support. Developing self-awareness, communicating effectively, setting boundaries, managing emotional reactions, seeking support, building trust gradually, and focusing on self-care are all essential components of successful relationship management. Remember that progress takes time, and it's okay to seek help along the way. By working on these skills, individuals with BPD can create more stable and satisfying relationships, enhancing their overall quality of life.

How BPD affects relationships and strategies for healthier interactions.

Borderline Personality Disorder (BPD) profoundly affects relationships due to its impact on emotions, behaviour, and self-perception. Understanding these effects and employing strategies for healthier interactions can help individuals with BPD build more stable and fulfilling relationships.

Impact of BPD on Relationships

1. Emotional Instability

   - Intense Emotions: Individuals with BPD often experience intense, rapidly changing emotions that can lead to unpredictable behaviour.

   - Impact: This emotional volatility can strain relationships, causing confusion and frustration for both parties.

2. Fear of Abandonment

- Overwhelming Fear: A pervasive fear of
abandonment can lead to clinginess or excessive
reassurance-seeking.

- Impact: This fear can cause tension and conflict, as
partners may feel overwhelmed by the constant need for
validation.

3. Black-and-White Thinking (Splitting)

- All-or-Nothing Perception: People with BPD may see
others as either all good or all bad, leading to idealisation
or devaluation.

- Impact: This can result in unstable relationships, as
someone may quickly go from being viewed as perfect
to being seen as entirely flawed.

4. Impulsivity

- Impulsive Behaviours: Impulsivity can lead to risky behaviours, such as substance abuse, spending sprees, or unsafe sexual activities.

- Impact: These behaviours can create instability and conflict in relationships, often damaging trust.

5. Identity Disturbance

- Unstable Self-Image: Inconsistent self-perception can affect how individuals relate to others and perceive their relationships.

- Impact: This can lead to difficulties in maintaining a consistent, stable connection with others.

Strategies for Healthier Interactions

1. Develop Emotional Regulation Skills

- Mindfulness: Practice mindfulness to become aware of your emotions without judgment. This helps in recognising and managing intense emotions before they escalate.

- DBT Techniques: Use Dialectical Behaviour Therapy (DBT) skills, such as distress tolerance and emotion regulation techniques, to handle emotional ups and downs effectively.

2. Improve Communication

- "I" Statements: Use "I" statements to express your feelings and needs clearly and without blame. For example, "I feel upset when..." instead of "You always make me feel..."

- Active Listening: Engage in active listening by fully concentrating on the speaker, understanding their message, and responding thoughtfully.

3. Set and Respect Boundaries

- Clarify Boundaries: Clearly define your boundaries and respect the boundaries of others. Communicate these boundaries openly to prevent misunderstandings.

- Practice Assertiveness: Use assertive communication to express your needs and boundaries without aggression. Techniques like DEAR MAN (Describe, Express, Assert, Reinforce, Mindful, Appear Confident, Negotiate) can be helpful.

4. Manage Fear of Abandonment

- Self-Validation: Practice self-validation to reduce dependence on external reassurance. Remind yourself of your worth and capabilities.

- Build Trust Gradually: Allow trust to develop slowly in relationships. Engage in small acts of trust and increase them as the relationship progresses.

5. Address Black-and-White Thinking

- Challenge Cognitive Distortions: Recognise and challenge all-or-nothing thinking patterns. Try to see people and situations in more balanced terms.

- Seek Multiple Perspectives: Get feedback from trusted friends or therapists to gain different perspectives on your thoughts and feelings.

6. Manage Impulsivity

- Pause Before Acting: When feeling impulsive, take a moment to pause and consider the potential consequences of your actions.

- Develop Coping Strategies: Identify and practice healthier coping mechanisms, such as exercise, creative activities, or talking to a friend, to manage impulsive urges.

7. Enhance Self-Awareness and Identity

  - Explore Your Interests: Engage in activities that reflect your interests and values to develop a stronger sense of self.

  - Therapeutic Support: Work with a therapist to explore and stabilise your self-identity. Therapy can provide a safe space to understand and accept yourself.

Supporting a Loved One with BPD

For partners, friends, and family members, supporting someone with BPD can be challenging but rewarding. Here are some tips for providing effective support:

1. Educate Yourself: Learn about BPD to better understand the challenges your loved one faces and how you can support them.

2. Be Patient and Compassionate: Recognise that their behaviours are symptoms of the disorder, not personal attacks. Offer empathy and patience.

3. Encourage Treatment: Support your loved one in seeking and adhering to treatment, such as therapy or medication, which can significantly improve their symptoms.

4. Set Healthy Boundaries: Maintain your well-being by setting and respecting boundaries. Ensure you have time for self-care and seek support if needed.

Navigating relationships with borderline personality disorder can be complex, but with understanding and effective strategies, it is possible to build healthier, more stable connections. By developing emotional regulation skills, improving communication, setting boundaries, managing fears, and seeking therapeutic support, individuals with BPD can enhance their relationships and overall quality of life. For loved ones, education, patience, and empathy are key to providing meaningful support. Together, these efforts can lead to more fulfilling and resilient relationships.

Chapter 8.

Self-Care and Well-being

- Importance of self-care practices and developing a routine that supports mental health.

Self-Care and Well-being

Borderline Personality Disorder (BPD) presents unique challenges that can significantly impact daily life, emotional well-being, and relationships. Effective self-care is crucial for managing symptoms, reducing stress, and enhancing overall quality of life. Here, we explore essential self-care practices tailored to individuals with BPD to promote emotional stability, mental health, and well-being.

Understanding the Importance of Self-Care in BPD

Self-care is not just about pampering oneself; it is about adopting habits and practices that support mental, emotional, and physical health. For those with BPD, self-care is a vital component of managing the disorder and leading a balanced life. It involves recognising personal needs, setting healthy boundaries, and engaging in activities that foster well-being.

Key Self-Care Strategies for BPD

1. Emotional Regulation and Mindfulness

- Practice Mindfulness:

- Technique: Engage in mindfulness exercises such as breath awareness, body scans, and mindful walking. These practices help increase present-moment awareness and reduce emotional reactivity.

- Benefits: Mindfulness can improve emotional regulation, decrease stress, and enhance self-awareness, making it easier to manage intense emotions.

- Use DBT Skills:

- Technique: Incorporate Dialectical Behaviour Therapy (DBT) skills into daily life. Skills like distress tolerance, emotion regulation, and interpersonal effectiveness are particularly useful.

- Benefits: DBT skills provide practical tools for managing crises, regulating emotions, and improving relationships, contributing to overall well-being.

2. Physical Self-Care

- Maintain a Healthy Lifestyle:

- Technique: Engage in regular physical activity, eat a balanced diet, and get adequate sleep. Avoid substances that can negatively impact your mood and health, such as alcohol and drugs.

- Benefits: Physical health directly influences mental health. Regular exercise, nutritious food, and proper sleep can improve mood, reduce anxiety, and increase energy levels.

- Relaxation Techniques:

- Technique: Practice relaxation techniques such as yoga, progressive muscle relaxation, or deep breathing exercises.

- Benefits: These techniques can reduce physical tension, lower stress levels, and promote a sense of calm and relaxation.

3. Mental Self-Care

- Therapeutic Support:

  - Technique: Engage in regular therapy sessions, whether individual, group, or family therapy. Therapists can provide support, strategies, and guidance tailored to your needs.

  - Benefits: Therapy can help you understand and manage BPD symptoms, work through past trauma, and develop healthier coping mechanisms.

- Engage in Hobbies and Interests:

  - Technique: Dedicate time to activities and hobbies that bring you joy and fulfilment, such as reading, painting, playing an instrument, or gardening.

  - Benefits: Engaging in enjoyable activities can distract from negative thoughts, boost mood, and provide a sense of accomplishment and purpose.

4. Social Self-Care

- Build a Support Network:

- Technique: Surround yourself with supportive, understanding individuals who respect your boundaries and encourage your well-being. This can include friends, family, support groups, or online communities.

- Benefits: A strong support network provides emotional support, reduces feelings of isolation, and offers practical assistance during difficult times.

- Communicate Effectively:

- Technique: Practice clear and assertive communication. Use "I" statements to express your feelings and needs, and actively listen to others.

- Benefits: Effective communication can improve relationships, reduce misunderstandings, and foster a supportive and respectful environment.

5. Spiritual Self-Care

- Explore Spiritual Practices:

- Technique: Engage in spiritual practices that resonate with you, such as meditation, prayer, or spending time in nature.

- Benefits: Spiritual practices can provide a sense of peace, purpose, and connection, enhancing overall well-being and resilience.

- Reflect on Values and Beliefs:

- Technique: Spend time reflecting on your values, beliefs, and what gives your life meaning. Journaling or discussing these with a trusted individual can be helpful.

- Benefits: Understanding your values and beliefs can guide your decisions, provide direction, and contribute to a more fulfilling life.

Incorporating Self-Care into Daily Life

1. Create a Self-Care Plan:

- Develop a personalised self-care plan that includes activities and practices tailored to your needs and preferences. Schedule these activities regularly and make them a non-negotiable part of your routine.

2. Set Realistic Goals:

- Set achievable and specific self-care goals. Start with small, manageable steps and gradually increase the complexity and duration of your self-care activities.

3. Monitor Progress:

  - Keep a self-care journal to track your activities, emotions, and progress. Reflect on what works well and what needs adjustment to optimise your self-care routine.

4. Seek Support:

  - Don't hesitate to seek support from therapists, support groups, or loved ones when implementing and maintaining your self-care practices. External support can provide motivation and accountability.

5. Be Kind to Yourself:

  - Practice self-compassion and kindness. Recognise that self-care is a journey, and it's okay to have setbacks. Celebrate your efforts and progress, no matter how small.

Self-care is a critical component of managing borderline personality disorder and enhancing overall well-being. By incorporating emotional regulation, physical health, mental support, social connections, and spiritual practices into daily life, individuals with BPD can create a balanced and fulfilling self-care routine. Remember, self-care is an ongoing process that requires patience, commitment, and flexibility. With consistent practice and support, self-care can lead to greater emotional stability, improved relationships, and a higher quality of life.

Importance of self-care practices and developing a routine that supports mental health.

Borderline Personality Disorder (BPD) is characterised by intense emotions, unstable relationships, and impulsive behaviours, making everyday life challenging for those affected. One of the most effective ways to manage BPD symptoms and enhance overall well-being is through consistent self-care practices. Developing a self-care routine tailored to support mental health can provide stability, improve emotional regulation, and foster a sense of control and balance.

Why Self-Care is Crucial in BPD

1. Emotional Regulation

- Impact: Individuals with BPD often experience intense, rapidly changing emotions that can be difficult to manage.

- Self-Care Role: Regular self-care practices, such as mindfulness and relaxation techniques, help regulate emotions and reduce the intensity of mood swings.

2. Stress Reduction

- Impact: Chronic stress can exacerbate BPD symptoms, leading to increased anxiety, depression, and emotional volatility.

- Self-Care Role: Engaging in stress-reducing activities like exercise, hobbies, and adequate rest can mitigate the impact of stress on mental health.

3. Improved Relationships

- Impact: BPD can strain relationships due to fears of abandonment, impulsivity, and emotional instability.

- Self-Care Role: By prioritising self-care, individuals can approach relationships with more stability and clarity, improving communication and connection with others.

4. Enhanced Self-Esteem and Self-Worth

- Impact: Many individuals with BPD struggle with low self-esteem and a fluctuating sense of self.

- Self-Care Role Self-care practices reinforce the importance of self-worth and self-respect, fostering a more positive self-image.

Developing a Self-Care Routine

Creating a consistent self-care routine tailored to individual needs is essential for managing BPD. Here's how to develop a routine that supports mental health:

1. Identify Personal Needs and Preferences

- Assessment: Reflect on what activities and practices make you feel calm, happy, and centred. Consider physical, emotional, mental, social, and spiritual needs.

- Personalisation: Tailor your self-care routine to include a mix of activities that address these areas.

2. Incorporate Emotional and Mental Self-Care

- Mindfulness and Meditation: Regular mindfulness practices, such as meditation, deep breathing exercises, and body scans, can help increase emotional awareness and reduce reactivity.

- Journaling: Keeping a journal to track emotions, thoughts, and experiences can provide insight and help process feelings.

- Therapy: Regular sessions with a therapist can provide support, strategies, and a safe space to explore and manage BPD symptoms.

3. Prioritise Physical Self-Care

- Exercise: Engage in regular physical activity that you enjoy, such as walking, dancing, yoga, or swimming. Exercise releases endorphins, which improve mood and reduce stress.

- Nutrition: Maintain a balanced diet rich in fruits, vegetables, whole grains, and lean proteins. Proper nutrition supports overall mental and physical health.

- Sleep: Establish a consistent sleep routine, aiming for 7-9 hours of sleep per night. Good sleep hygiene includes a regular bedtime, a calming pre-sleep routine, and a comfortable sleep environment.

4. Engage in Social and Recreational Activities

   - Support Network: Build and maintain a supportive network of friends, family, or support groups. Regular social interactions can provide emotional support and reduce feelings of isolation.

   - Hobbies: Dedicate time to hobbies and interests that bring joy and fulfilment. Engaging in creative or recreational activities can be a healthy outlet for stress and emotions.

5. Incorporate Relaxation and Stress-Reduction Techniques

   - Relaxation Practices: Include activities like reading, listening to music, taking baths, or spending time in nature to unwind and relax.

   - Mind-Body Practices: Techniques such as yoga, tai chi, or progressive muscle relaxation can help reduce physical and mental tension.

6. Set Realistic Goals and Track Progress

   - Goal Setting: Set achievable self-care goals and gradually increase the complexity and duration of activities as you build confidence and routine.

   - Monitoring: Use a self-care journal or app to track your activities, emotions, and progress. Reflect on what works well and make adjustments as needed.

7. Practice Self-Compassion

   - Self-Kindness: Treat yourself with kindness and understanding, especially during setbacks. Recognise that self-care is an ongoing journey, not a destination.

   - Positive Affirmations: Use positive affirmations to reinforce self-worth and resilience. Remind yourself of your strengths and achievements regularly.

For individuals with borderline personality disorder, self-care is a vital component of managing symptoms and improving quality of life. By developing a consistent self-care routine that includes emotional, mental, physical, social, and relaxation practices, individuals can gain greater control over their emotions, reduce stress, and enhance their overall well-being. Remember, self-care is a personal journey that requires patience, dedication, and flexibility. With commitment and the right strategies, self-care can become a powerful tool in navigating life with BPD, leading to a more balanced, stable, and fulfilling existence.

Chapter 9.

Setting Boundaries

- Learning to set and maintain boundaries to protect emotional well-being.

Setting Boundaries

Borderline Personality Disorder (BPD) is often characterised by intense emotions, fear of abandonment, and difficulties in maintaining stable relationships. One of the most essential skills for managing BPD and fostering healthier relationships is setting and maintaining boundaries. Boundaries help protect emotional well-being, reduce stress, and enhance interpersonal interactions. Here's a guide on why boundaries are crucial and how to set them effectively when dealing with BPD.

Why Boundaries Matter in BPD

1. Emotional Protection

- Impact: Individuals with BPD are often more sensitive to emotional stimuli and can become overwhelmed easily.

- Boundaries Role: Boundaries act as a buffer, protecting against emotional overload and helping to manage intense feelings.

2. Relationship Stability

- Impact: BPD can lead to turbulent relationships marked by extreme closeness and sudden distancing.

- Boundaries Role: Clear boundaries provide structure and predictability in relationships, reducing conflict and fostering stability.

3. Self-Identity

- Impact: BPD often involves an unstable sense of self and difficulty understanding personal limits and needs.

- Boundaries Role: Setting boundaries helps individuals with BPD define their identity, preferences, and values, contributing to a more stable self-concept.

4. Empowerment and Control

- Impact: Feelings of helplessness and loss of control are common in BPD.

- Boundaries Role: Establishing boundaries empowers individuals to take control of their interactions and environment, promoting a sense of agency.

Strategies for Setting Boundaries

1. Self-Awareness and Reflection

- Identify Needs: Reflect on your emotional and physical needs. Consider what makes you feel safe, respected, and valued.

- Recognise Limits: Understand your limits in various aspects of life, including work, relationships, and personal space.

2. Communicate Clearly and Assertively

- Use "I" Statements: Express your boundaries using "I" statements, such as "I need time alone after work to relax" or "I feel uncomfortable when you raise your voice."

- Be Direct and Specific: Clearly articulate what your boundaries are and why they are important. Avoid vague language to prevent misunderstandings.

3. Practice Consistency

- Enforce Boundaries: Consistently uphold your boundaries. If you've set a boundary about needing alone time, stick to it even if it feels challenging.

- Reinforce Respectfully: Remind others of your boundaries if they are crossed. Use respectful and calm communication to reinforce your needs.

4. Manage Fear of Rejection

- Acknowledge Fears: Recognise that fear of rejection or abandonment may arise when setting boundaries. Understand that these feelings are valid but do not have to dictate your actions.

- Build Trust Gradually: Trust that respecting your boundaries will lead to healthier relationships. People who care about you will respect your needs and limits.

5. Use Support Systems

- Seek Guidance: Talk to a therapist or counsellor about your challenges with setting boundaries. They can provide strategies and support tailored to your needs.

- Lean on Trusted Individuals: Discuss your boundaries with trusted friends or family members who can support you and hold you accountable.

6. Implement Self-Care

- Prioritise Well-Being: Ensure that your boundaries reflect a commitment to your well-being. Self-care activities, such as exercise, hobbies, and relaxation, should be non-negotiable.

- Reflect and Adjust: Regularly reflect on how your boundaries are impacting your mental health and relationships. Adjust them as necessary to ensure they continue to serve your needs.

7. Deal with Pushback

- Stay Firm: When others push back against your boundaries, stay firm and calm. Reiterate your needs and the importance of respecting them.

- Evaluate Relationships: If someone consistently disrespects your boundaries, it may be necessary to reevaluate the relationship and consider distancing yourself from them.

Examples of Healthy Boundaries

1. Emotional Boundaries

- "I need time to process my emotions before discussing this topic."

- "I am not comfortable discussing this personal issue right now."

2. Physical Boundaries

- "I need personal space to feel comfortable."

- "I prefer not to be touched without asking first."

3. Time Boundaries

- "I need to leave social events by 10 PM to get enough rest."

- "I can't take on extra work this weekend; I need time to recharge."

4. Social Boundaries

- "I need to limit our conversations about negative news as it affects my mental health."

- "I prefer one-on-one interactions over group settings."

Setting boundaries is a crucial skill for individuals with borderline personality disorder to maintain emotional well-being, foster stable relationships, and support self-identity. By developing self-awareness, communicating clearly, and practicing consistency, individuals can create boundaries that protect their mental health and enhance their quality of life. Remember, setting boundaries is not about building walls but about defining spaces where you can thrive. With patience, practice, and support, boundary-setting can become a powerful tool for navigating life with BPD.

Learning to set and maintain boundaries to protect emotional well-being.

Borderline Personality Disorder (BPD) can make navigating personal relationships and managing emotions particularly challenging. One of the most effective strategies for maintaining emotional well-being is learning to set and maintain healthy boundaries. Boundaries help define personal limits, protect emotional space, and promote stability in interactions with others. Here's a guide on how individuals with BPD can develop and sustain boundaries to safeguard their mental health.

The Importance of Boundaries in BPD

1. Emotional Safety

   - Impact: People with BPD often experience heightened sensitivity to emotional triggers and can become overwhelmed easily.

- Role of Boundaries: Boundaries create a safe space where individuals can process emotions without external pressures, reducing the likelihood of emotional overload.

2. Relationship Stability

- Impact: BPD can lead to tumultuous relationships due to fears of abandonment, intense emotions, and impulsive behaviours.

- Role of Boundaries: Clear boundaries provide structure and predictability, helping to stabilise relationships and reduce conflict.

3. Self-Respect and Identity

- Impact: Individuals with BPD may struggle with an unstable sense of self and difficulty asserting their needs.

- Role of Boundaries: Setting boundaries reinforces self-respect and helps define personal values and identity.

4. Stress Reduction

- Impact: Stress can exacerbate BPD symptoms, leading to increased emotional instability.

- Role of Boundaries: Boundaries help manage and reduce stress by preventing overcommitment and ensuring personal needs are met.

Steps to Setting and Maintaining Boundaries

1. Understand Your Needs and Limits

- Self-Reflection: Spend time reflecting on your emotional, physical, and mental needs. Identify what makes you feel safe, respected, and valued.

- Recognise Triggers: Be aware of situations or behaviours that trigger intense emotions or stress, and consider how boundaries can mitigate these triggers.

2. Communicate Clearly and Assertively

- Use "I" Statements: Express your boundaries using "I" statements to emphasise your feelings and needs. For example, "I feel overwhelmed when there's too much noise, so I need some quiet time."

- Be Specific: Clearly articulate your boundaries and the reasons behind them. Specificity helps prevent misunderstandings and ensures your needs are understood.

3. Practice Consistency

- Enforce Boundaries: Consistently uphold your boundaries even when it feels challenging. If you've set a boundary about needing alone time, honour it consistently.

- Reinforce Boundaries Respectfully: If someone crosses your boundary, remind them calmly and respectfully. Consistent reinforcement helps others understand and respect your limits.

4. Manage Fear of Rejection

- Acknowledge Fears: Recognise that setting boundaries may evoke fears of rejection or abandonment. Understand that these feelings are valid but should not deter you from maintaining your boundaries.

- Trust in Respect: Believe that respecting your boundaries will lead to healthier and more respectful relationships. Those who care about you will honour your needs.

5. Use Support Systems

- Seek Professional Guidance: Work with a therapist or counsellor to develop boundary-setting skills. They can provide tailored strategies and support.

- Lean on Trusted Individuals: Discuss your boundaries with trusted friends or family members who can offer support and accountability.

6. Incorporate Self-Care

- Prioritise Well-Being: Ensure your boundaries reflect a commitment to your well-being. Engage in regular self-care activities that nurture your mental, emotional, and physical health.

- Reflect and Adjust: Regularly assess how your boundaries impact your well-being and relationships. Adjust them as necessary to ensure they continue to serve your needs.

Examples of Healthy Boundaries

1. Emotional Boundaries

- "I need time to process my emotions before discussing this topic."

- "I'm not comfortable talking about this right now."

2. Physical Boundaries

   - "I need personal space to feel comfortable."

   - "Please ask before touching me."

3. Time Boundaries

   - "I need to leave events by 10 PM to get enough rest."

   - "I can't take on extra tasks this weekend; I need time to relax."

4. Social Boundaries

   - "I need to limit our conversations about negative news."

   - "I prefer smaller gatherings over large groups."

Dealing with Pushback

1. Stay Firm

- Consistency: When others push back against your boundaries, remain firm and calm. Reiterate your needs clearly and confidently.

- Self-Validation: Remind yourself why your boundaries are important and validate your right to maintain them.

2. Evaluate Relationships

- Assess Respect: If someone consistently disrespects your boundaries, it may be necessary to reevaluate the relationship and consider distancing yourself from them.

- Seek Support: Talk to a therapist or trusted individual about how to handle persistent boundary violations.

Setting and maintaining boundaries is a critical skill for individuals with borderline personality disorder to protect emotional well-being and foster healthier relationships. By understanding personal needs, communicating clearly, practicing consistency, and seeking support, individuals can create and sustain boundaries that enhance their mental health and stability. Remember, boundaries are not about isolating oneself but about creating a safe and respectful space where one can thrive. With patience, practice, and determination, boundary-setting can become a powerful tool in managing BPD and leading a balanced, fulfilling life.

Chapter 10.

Personal Growth and Recovery

- Stories of hope, resilience, and personal growth from individuals with BPD.

Finding Light at the End of the Tunnel: Hope and Help for Those with BPD

Personal Growth and Recovery

Borderline Personality Disorder (BPD) presents unique challenges that can profoundly impact daily life, relationships, and self-perception. However, personal growth and recovery are possible with the right mindset, strategies, and support. Embracing the journey toward stability and fulfilment involves understanding BPD, committing to self-improvement, and nurturing resilience. Here's a guide on how individuals with BPD can foster personal growth and achieve recovery.

Understanding BPD and the Recovery Journey

1. Acknowledging the Diagnosis

- Impact: Receiving a BPD diagnosis can be overwhelming, but it's the first step toward understanding and managing the disorder.

- Acceptance: Accepting the diagnosis allows individuals to address their symptoms, seek appropriate treatments, and embark on a path to recovery.

2. Setting Realistic Expectations

- Impact: Recovery from BPD is not linear and involves ongoing effort and commitment.

- Patience: Recognise that progress may be gradual. Celebrate small achievements and be patient with setbacks.

Key Components of Personal Growth and Recovery

1. Therapeutic Support

- Individual Therapy: Engaging in therapy, such as Dialectical Behaviour Therapy (DBT), can provide tools for managing emotions, improving relationships, and reducing self-destructive behaviours.

- Group Therapy: Participating in group therapy offers support from others who understand BPD, fostering a sense of community and shared experience.

2. Developing Coping Skills

  - Emotion Regulation: Learn techniques to manage intense emotions, such as mindfulness, deep breathing, and grounding exercises.

  - Distress Tolerance: Develop skills to cope with crisis without resorting to harmful behaviours. Techniques include distraction, self-soothing, and reality acceptance.

3. Building a Support Network

  - Trusted Relationships: Surround yourself with understanding and supportive individuals who respect your boundaries and encourage your growth.

  - Peer Support: Engage with support groups or online communities where you can share experiences and gain insights from others facing similar challenges.

4. Establishing Healthy Boundaries

  - Self-Respect: Learn to set and maintain boundaries that protect your emotional well-being. Clear boundaries help prevent emotional overload and maintain relationship stability.

- Assertive Communication: Practice communicating your needs and limits assertively and respectfully.

5. Prioritising Self-Care

- Physical Health: Engage in regular exercise, maintain a balanced diet, and ensure adequate sleep. Physical well-being supports mental health.

- Mental Health: Dedicate time to activities that promote relaxation and joy, such as hobbies, meditation, and spending time in nature.

6. Cultivating Self-Compassion

- Self-Kindness: Treat yourself with the same kindness and understanding you would offer a friend. Acknowledge your efforts and progress.

- Forgiveness: Forgive yourself for past mistakes and recognise that growth involves learning and evolving.

7. Setting Goals and Tracking Progress

 - Realistic Goals: Set achievable and specific goals that align with your recovery journey. Break them down into manageable steps.

 - Reflect and Adjust: Regularly review your progress, celebrate successes, and adjust your goals as needed. Keep a journal to track your journey and reflect on your experiences.

Overcoming Challenges in the Recovery Process

1. Managing Setbacks

 - Resilience: Understand that setbacks are a natural part of the recovery process. Use them as opportunities to learn and grow stronger.

 - Support: Reach out to your support network during difficult times. Professional guidance can provide additional strategies for overcoming challenges.

2. Navigating Relationships

   - Communication: Maintain open and honest communication with loved ones. Educate them about BPD to foster empathy and understanding.

   - Boundaries: Continue to enforce healthy boundaries to ensure your relationships are supportive and respectful.

3. Sustaining Motivation

   - Inspiration: Find inspiration in stories of others who have successfully managed BPD. Their journeys can provide hope and motivation.

   - Self-Reminders: Remind yourself of your reasons for pursuing recovery. Visualise the benefits of achieving your goals, such as improved relationships and emotional stability.

Personal growth and recovery with borderline personality disorder are attainable through dedication, self-awareness, and the right support. By embracing therapeutic techniques, developing coping skills, and building a robust support network, individuals with BPD can navigate their path to stability and fulfilment. Remember, recovery is a journey, not a destination. With patience, resilience, and self-compassion, it's possible to overcome the challenges of BPD and lead a balanced, rewarding life.

Stories of hope, resilience, and personal growth from individuals with BPD.

Borderline Personality Disorder (BPD) can be a challenging condition to manage, but many individuals have found ways to thrive despite their diagnosis. Their stories offer hope, resilience, and personal growth, inspiring others who face similar struggles. Here are some notable figures who have publicly shared their experiences with BPD, demonstrating that recovery and success are possible.

1. Emilia Clarke

Background: Emilia Clarke is an acclaimed actress best known for her role as Daenerys Targaryen on the hit television series "Game of Thrones."

Journey with BPD: Clarke has been open about her struggles with mental health, including severe anxiety and periods of depression. While she hasn't publicly confirmed a BPD diagnosis, her experiences with intense emotions and identity struggles resonate with those common in BPD.

Resilience and Growth: Clarke has used her platform to advocate for mental health awareness. She founded SameYou, a charity aimed at increasing rehabilitation access for young adults following brain injury and stroke, stemming from her own experiences with brain aneurysms. Her advocacy work and transparency about her mental health challenges inspire many to seek help and support.

2. Stephen Fry

Background: Stephen Fry is a beloved British actor, comedian, writer, and presenter, known for his wit and extensive work in film, television, and literature.

Journey with BPD: Fry has openly discussed his struggles with bipolar disorder, which often co-occurs with BPD and shares some overlapping symptoms such as mood instability and impulsivity. While not diagnosed with BPD, his experiences provide valuable insights into managing complex mental health conditions.

Resilience and Growth: Fry has been a vocal advocate for mental health awareness, sharing his journey through documentaries, interviews, and his autobiography. His openness has helped reduce the stigma surrounding mental illness and encouraged others to seek support. His contributions to mental health advocacy have been recognised and celebrated widely.

3. Pete Doherty

Background: Pete Doherty is a British musician and songwriter, best known as the frontman of The Libertines and Babyshambles.

Journey with BPD: Doherty has faced significant public and personal struggles with addiction and mental health issues. He has spoken about his battles with self-destructive behaviour and the intense emotions that have impacted his life and career. While he hasn't confirmed a BPD diagnosis, his experiences align with many symptoms of the disorder.

Resilience and Growth: Doherty's journey toward recovery has involved seeking professional help and making efforts to manage his mental health. His story serves as a testament to the challenges of living with a complex mental health condition and the possibility of finding a path to stability and creative expression.

4. Brandon Marshall

Background: Brandon Marshall is a former NFL wide receiver who has played for teams like the Denver Broncos, Miami Dolphins, and New York Jets.

Journey with BPD: In 2011, Brandon Marshall publicly revealed his BPD diagnosis. He faced difficulties with mood swings, impulsivity, and maintaining relationships. His decision to speak openly about his condition was driven by a desire to break the stigma surrounding mental health.

Resilience and Growth: Marshall sought treatment, including Dialectical Behaviour Therapy (DBT), which helped him manage his symptoms and improve his relationships. He also founded Project 375, an organisation dedicated to eradicating the stigma of mental illness and promoting mental health awareness. His advocacy work and transparency have provided hope to many struggling with similar issues.

5. Darrell Hammond

Background: Darrell Hammond is a comedian and actor best known for his work on "Saturday Night Live" (SNL), where he performed from 1995 to 2009.

Journey with BPD: Darrell Hammond has spoken candidly about his struggles with BPD, as well as other mental health challenges, including trauma and addiction. His symptoms were exacerbated by a difficult childhood, and for many years, he self-medicated to cope with his emotional pain.

Resilience and Growth: Hammond eventually sought professional help, which included therapy and medication. In his memoir, "God, If You're Not Up There, I'm F*cked," he details his journey toward healing and recovery. By sharing his story, Hammond has become an advocate for mental health, encouraging others to seek help and not suffer in silence.

6. AJ Mendez (AJ Lee)

Background: AJ Mendez, known professionally as AJ Lee, is a retired professional wrestler and author. She achieved fame in WWE (World Wrestling Entertainment) and is a three-time Divas Champion.

Journey with BPD: In her memoir, "Crazy Is My Superpower," AJ Mendez revealed her diagnosis of BPD and discussed the challenges she faced growing up with mental health issues, including depression and anxiety. Her journey included periods of self-harm and suicidal thoughts.

Resilience and Growth: Mendez's resilience is evident in her successful wrestling career and her ability to channel her struggles into strength. Her book has inspired many, particularly young women, by showing that it's possible to overcome mental health challenges and achieve one's dreams. She continues to be an advocate for mental health awareness.

7. Pete Davidson

Background: Pete Davidson is a comedian and actor, known for his work on "Saturday Night Live" and in various films.

Journey with BPD: Davidson has been open about his diagnosis of BPD, sharing that he has struggled with intense emotions, unstable relationships, and self-destructive behaviour. His transparency about his condition has brought attention to the realities of living with BPD.

Resilience and Growth: Davidson sought treatment, including therapy and medication, which has helped him manage his symptoms. He uses his platform to discuss mental health openly, reducing stigma and encouraging others to seek help. His humour and candidness about his struggles have made him a relatable and inspiring figure for many.

8. Martha Wainwright

Background: Martha Wainwright is a singer-songwriter from a famous musical family, including her brother Rufus Wainwright and parents Loudon Wainwright III and Kate McGarrigle.

Journey with BPD: Wainwright has discussed her diagnosis of BPD and how it has influenced her life and music. She has experienced the intense emotions and relationship difficulties characteristic of the disorder.

Resilience and Growth: Through therapy and her music, Wainwright has found ways to cope with her BPD. Her songs often reflect her emotional struggles and journey towards understanding and managing her condition. Her openness about her mental health has helped fans who face similar issues feel less alone.

The stories of these people are in the spotlight and demonstrate that it is possible to lead a fulfilling and successful life despite a diagnosis of borderline personality disorder. Their journeys of hope, resilience, and personal growth serve as powerful reminders that seeking help, embracing treatment, and advocating for mental health can lead to positive outcomes. These individuals inspire others to face their challenges head-on and believe in the possibility of recovery and personal growth.

Finding Light at the End of the Tunnel: Hope and Help for Those with BPD

Living with Borderline Personality Disorder (BPD) can sometimes feel like navigating a stormy sea, where emotions surge and crash, making it difficult to see a clear path ahead. However, it's essential to remember that there is help available, and many have found their way to calmer waters. There is light at the end of the tunnel for those with BPD, and with the right support and strategies, a fulfilling and stable life is within reach.

Understanding BPD

BPD is a complex mental health condition characterised by intense emotions, unstable relationships, and impulsive behaviours. It's often accompanied by a deep fear of abandonment and a fluctuating self-image. These symptoms can make daily life challenging, but they do not define you. With awareness and understanding, you can learn to manage BPD effectively.

Seeking Professional Help

One of the most crucial steps towards recovery is seeking professional help. Therapists, counsellors, and psychiatrists are trained to support individuals with BPD. They can provide a diagnosis, develop a treatment plan, and offer therapies that are specifically designed to address the symptoms of BPD. Dialectical Behaviour Therapy (DBT) is one such therapy that has shown significant effectiveness in treating BPD. DBT teaches skills for emotion regulation, distress tolerance, interpersonal effectiveness, and mindfulness.

Building a Support System

No one should have to face BPD alone. Building a strong support system of friends, family, and peers who understand and respect your experiences can provide immense comfort and encouragement. Support groups, both in-person and online, can also offer a sense of community and shared understanding. Connecting with others who have similar experiences can help you feel less isolated and more hopeful about the future.

Developing Coping Skills

Learning and practicing coping skills can make a significant difference in managing BPD. Techniques such as mindfulness, grounding exercises, and self-soothing strategies can help you stay present and calm during emotional storms. Setting and maintaining healthy boundaries is also vital for protecting your emotional well-being and fostering stable relationships.

Embracing Self-Care

Prioritising self-care is essential for managing BPD and promoting overall well-being. Engage in activities that bring you joy and relaxation, whether it's reading, painting, exercising, or spending time in nature. Regular self-care routines help reduce stress, improve mood, and enhance your ability to cope with challenges.

Celebrating Progress

Recovery from BPD is not a linear journey, and it's essential to celebrate your progress, no matter how small. Each step forward, whether it's attending a therapy session, practicing a new coping skill, or setting a boundary, is a victory. Recognise your efforts and give yourself credit for the hard work you're putting into your recovery.

Inspiring Stories of Hope

Many people with BPD have found their way to stability and fulfilment, and their stories offer hope and inspiration. Public figures like Brandon Marshall, Darrell Hammond, and AJ Mendez have shared their experiences with BPD, demonstrating that recovery is possible. They have used their platforms to advocate for mental health awareness, reduce stigma, and encourage others to seek help.

Moving Forward with Hope

Living with BPD can be incredibly challenging, but it's important to remember that you are not alone, and help is available. By seeking professional support, building a strong support network, developing coping skills, and prioritising self-care, you can navigate the complexities of BPD and move toward a brighter future.

There is light at the end of the tunnel. With patience, persistence, and support, you can find your way through the storm and into a life filled with hope, stability, and fulfilment. Remember, your journey is unique, and every step you take is a testament to your strength and resilience. Keep moving forward, and know that a better tomorrow is possible.